DEBORAH MEYERS

Macro Power: Unlock Your Potential

Mastering Macronutrients: Understanding, Implementing, and Maximizing the Benefits

This book was professionally typeset on Reedsy.
Find out more at reedsy.com

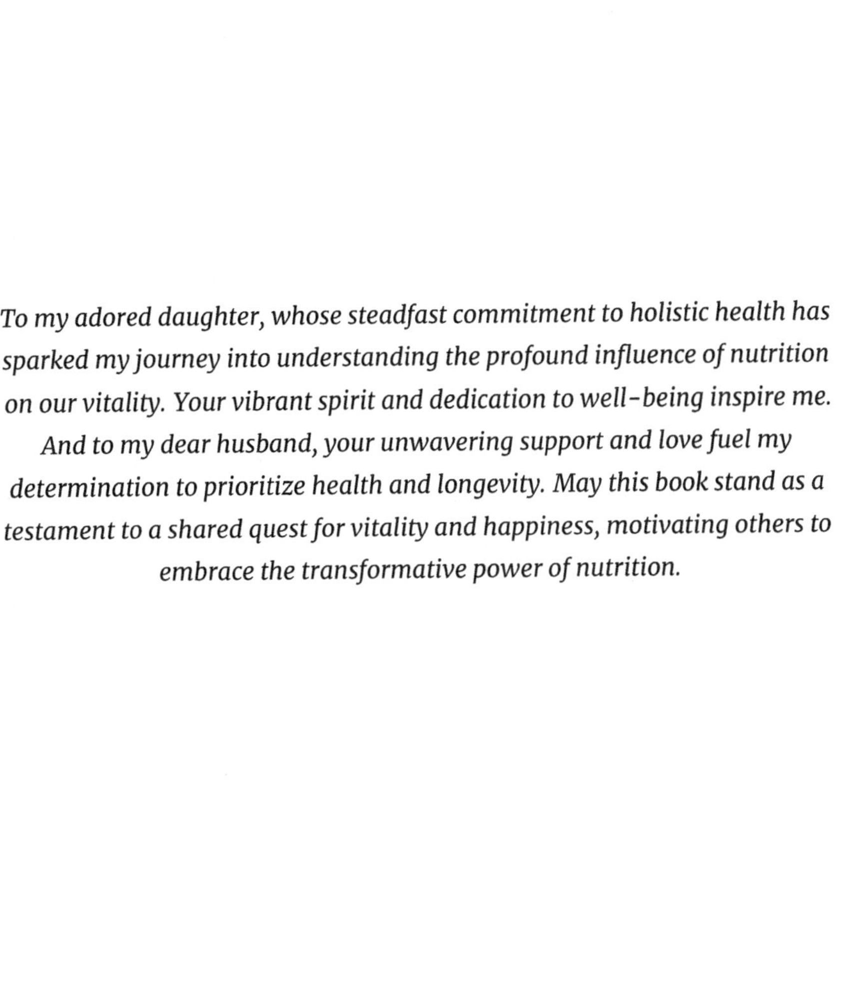

To my adored daughter, whose steadfast commitment to holistic health has sparked my journey into understanding the profound influence of nutrition on our vitality. Your vibrant spirit and dedication to well–being inspire me. And to my dear husband, your unwavering support and love fuel my determination to prioritize health and longevity. May this book stand as a testament to a shared quest for vitality and happiness, motivating others to embrace the transformative power of nutrition.

"In the end, it's not just about adding years to our lives, but about adding life to our years."

- Unknown

Contents

1

Introduction

I suspect you are picking up this book because you have been hearing more and more about counting macros or macronutrients. Counting macros has become popular among those looking to lose weight and gain muscle.

You may have seen references on your social media feeds, or it's been a discussion topic in the hallways at work or social engagements. When searching the internet for diet, weight loss, or macros, you can be overwhelmed with information, which can be confusing. If you have experience counting calories and are familiar with macros, you might be intimidated at the thought of having to do mathematical calculations. Rest assured, you can do this.

One of the pitfalls of starting a sustainable diet plan is choosing between many options. Let's face it: You can jump on an all-meat/high-protein plan, vegetarian or plant-based, low-carbohydrate, no-fat plan, etc. You can also take the problem-solving approach and pursue anti-inflammation, balancing hormones, burning fat, or healing metabolism—and I've just named a few.

There is a lot of information out there which isn't always straightforward. This book provides the fundamental facts to help you learn what you need to know and feel confident about doing so. By the end of this book, you will have a solid understanding of macronutrients, why they are essential, how to implement a plan, and how to maximize long-term sustainability benefits.

Let's dive in!

2

What are Macronutrients?

L et's first start by hitting the reset button. Our bodies need nutrition. Nutrition can not only sustain us but can improve the *quality* of our lives. Food variety provides the nutrients our bodies need. You don't get the same nutrients from a slice of bread as a steak or a handful of blueberries. When you narrow your intake to a select food group, as with some restrictive diets, you essentially starve yourself of those other vital nutrients. You could be undernourished. A balanced diet includes a variety of foods from the various nutrient groups.

Nutritional scientists have covered much ground on the varying intake rates of essential nutrients and their impact on body functions; however, let's save the scientific reports for graduate students. Most people want to have energy throughout the day, feel good in their clothes, be able to take a hike or spend hours exploring that special vacation spot, and sleep well (oh, and a regular BM, please).

Your body uses three nutrients, called macronutrients (or macros), for optimal functioning: carbohydrates, proteins, and fats. These macronutrients provide your body with energy in the form of calories. Calorie-restrictive diets are popular, and many applications on the market assist you in tracking calorie counts. The challenge with calorie counting alone as a focus in diet and weight loss is that not all calories are equal in their nutritional value or the "job" they perform in your body.

Your body's energy mainly comes from carbohydrates, while proteins help to build and repair body tissue. Fats help you feel full and help with the absorption of other vitamins and minerals. You can quickly gain weight if you count calories alone, and most of your calories come from simple carbohydrates (baked goods like bread, table sugar, and milk).

3

Carbohydrates

There are simple and complex carbohydrates, but the main difference is how quickly they are absorbed by the body.

Importance of Carbohydrates

1. Energy Source: Carbohydrates are the body's primary source of energy. When consumed, carbohydrates are broken down into glucose, which cells use as fuel for various metabolic processes. Glucose is essential for high-intensity activities and brain function.
2. Brain Function: The brain relies heavily on glucose for energy. Consuming an adequate amount of carbohydrates ensures proper cognitive function, concentration, and mental clarity.
3. Muscle Fuel: Carbohydrates provide energy for muscles during physical activity. Glycogen, the storage form of glucose in muscles, is a readily available fuel source during exercise, helping to sustain endurance and performance.
4. Metabolic Regulation: Carbohydrates play a role in metabolic regulation, particularly insulin production and blood sugar control. Fiber-rich carbohydrates can help stabilize blood sugar levels and

reduce the risk of insulin resistance and type 2 diabetes.

5. Digestive Health: Certain carbohydrates, such as dietary fiber, promote digestive health by adding bulk to stool, regulating bowel movements, and supporting the growth of beneficial gut bacteria. Adequate fiber intake is associated with a lower risk of constipation, diverticulosis, and colon cancer.

Common Misconceptions

1. Carbohydrates Cause Weight Gain: One of the most prevalent misconceptions is that consuming carbohydrates leads to weight gain. While excessive intake of refined carbohydrates and sugary foods can contribute to weight gain, not all carbohydrates are created equal. Whole, unprocessed carbohydrates like fruits, vegetables, whole grains, and legumes are nutrient-dense. They can be part of a healthy diet.

2. Carbohydrates are Unhealthy: Some people believe that carbohydrates are inherently unhealthy and should be avoided. However, carbohydrates are essential nutrients that provide energy and nutrients like vitamins, minerals, and phytonutrients (plant-producing compounds, antioxidants). The key is to choose complex carbohydrates from whole food sources rather than refined and processed options.

3. Carbohydrates Are Always High in Sugar: While some carbohydrates, such as table sugar and sugary beverages, are high in refined sugars, not all carbohydrates are. Complex carbohydrates in whole grains, fruits, and vegetables contain natural sugars, fiber, vitamins, and minerals, providing a more balanced nutritional profile.

Foods to Eat

1. Whole Grains: Opt for whole grains like oats, quinoa, brown rice, barley, whole wheat bread, and pasta. These foods are rich in complex carbohydrates, fiber, and nutrients, providing sustained energy and promoting satiety.
2. Fruits: Enjoy a variety of fruits, such as berries, apples, oranges, bananas, and melons. Fruits are excellent sources of natural sugars, vitamins, minerals, and antioxidants, making them nutritious choices for snacks or desserts.
3. Vegetables: Eat a colorful array of vegetables, including leafy greens, cruciferous vegetables, tomatoes, peppers, carrots, and sweet potatoes. Vegetables are low in calories and rich in fiber, vitamins, minerals, and phytonutrients, supporting overall health and well-being.
4. Legumes: incorporate beans, lentils, chickpeas, and peas into your meals. Legumes are high in fiber, protein, complex carbohydrates, and various nutrients, making them filling and nutritious additions to soups, salads, and main dishes.
5. Dairy: Choose dairy products like milk, yogurt, and kefir. These provide carbohydrates in the form of lactose, along with protein, calcium, and other essential nutrients. Opt for low-fat or non-fat varieties to reduce saturated fat intake.

By focusing on whole, nutrient-dense carbohydrates and balancing them with protein and healthy fats, you can optimize your diet for energy, health, and vitality.

Excess calories from *any* macronutrient can lead to weight gain. Our food and drink contain three types of carbohydrates: fiber, starches, and sugars. Fiber and starches are complex carbohydrates, and sugars are simple carbohydrates. The key is to choose complex carbohydrates (such as whole grains, fruits, and vegetables) over refined and sugary ones.

One of the most important carbohydrates is glucose. When you hear the term "blood sugar," it refers to glucose. Our cells use glucose for energy, and the brain is particularly dependent on it.

Carbohydrates are the most plentiful in our diets today and are the body's main fuel source. When you eat carbohydrates, they are broken down by your digestive system and absorbed into the bloodstream in the form of glucose, also known as blood sugar. Your body stores excess glucose in your muscles and liver, but once those stores are at the maximum, your body turns the extra glucose into fat. Given carbs turn to blood sugar, consuming too much can result in high blood sugar and increase your risk for diabetes.

Our body utilizes different types of carbohydrates for energy, storage, and structural purposes. Monosaccharides provide immediate energy, disaccharides break down into monosaccharides, and polysaccharides serve as energy stores and structural components. Including a variety in our diet ensures optimal health and function.

Monosaccharides

- Monosaccharides are the simplest form of carbohydrates. They consist of single sugar molecules. They are easy to digest and get into the blood.
- Examples include glucose, fructose, and galactose. Fructose is found in various fruits, such as grapes, pears, watermelon, and bananas. Galactose is found in milk products such as yogurt, cheese, and butter.
- Glucose is essential because it serves as the primary energy source for our cells. It's readily absorbed into the bloodstream and used for immediate energy while fructose can be absorbed slowly. Taken through a blood panel, the normal glucose level is 65–110 mg/dL.

Disaccharides

- Disaccharides are composed of two monosaccharide units linked together.
- Common disaccharides include:
- Sucrose: Composed of glucose and fructose. Found in table sugar and many sweet foods.
- Lactose: Composed of glucose and galactose. Found in milk and dairy products.
- Maltose: Composed of two glucose molecules. Found in malted foods and beverages. Malted foods are those that contain malt or malted barley as an ingredient. Malt is a product derived from sprouted barley grains that have been dried and sometimes roasted. It's commonly used as a sweetener and flavoring agent in various food and beverage products.
- Enzymes in our digestive system break down disaccharides into monosaccharides for absorption.

Polysaccharides

- Polysaccharides are complex carbohydrates made up of long chains of monosaccharide units.
- They serve as storage forms of energy and provide structural support.
- Examples of polysaccharides include:
- Starch: found in plant-based foods (such as grains, legumes, and tubers). Our body breaks down starch into glucose for energy.
- Glycogen: stored in our liver and muscles. When needed, it is broken down into glucose to maintain blood sugar levels.
- Cellulose: a major component of plant cell walls. Although we can't digest cellulose, it provides dietary fiber and supports digestive

health.

Dietary Fiber

- Dietary fiber is a carbohydrate found in plant-based foods like fruit, vegetables, and whole-grain products.
- Fiber is considered a complex healthy carbohydrate. It includes both soluble and insoluble fibers. Soluble fiber dissolves in water and forms a gel-like substance in the digestive tract, which helps to regulate blood sugar levels and lower cholesterol.
- Insoluble fiber cannot dissolve in water and adds bulk to stool, promoting regular bowel movements and preventing constipation.
- Fiber also helps you feel full longer and helps regulate blood sugar and lower cholesterol.

High-fiber foods include grains, legumes, tubers, root vegetables, and fruits. Wheat, rice, and corn are "grains;" beans, peas, and peanuts are "legumes;" potatoes are "tubers," and carrots and turnips are "root vegetables." Roots take in water, and tubers are considered part of the plant stem (not the root). Fruits include apples and peaches and vegetables like broccoli and Brussels sprouts.

4

Proteins

Some people believe that protein is only necessary for body-builders or athletes. Protein plays a crucial role in various bodily functions, including muscle repair, immune system support, and hormone production. While high-protein diets have gained popularity, they are only suitable for some. Excessive protein intake can strain kidneys and may not be necessary for sedentary individuals. When tracking macros, we emphasize balance in protein consumption based on *your* goals.

Importance of Protein

1. Muscle Health: Proteins are the building blocks of muscles. Adequate protein intake supports muscle growth, repair, and maintenance, which is crucial for staying active.
2. Cellular Function: Proteins play roles in various cellular functions, including enzyme production, immune system support, and hormone regulation. They're involved in virtually every biological process in the body.
3. Satiety and Weight Management: Protein-rich foods help you feel

more full than carbohydrates or fats. Consuming adequate protein can help curb appetite, reduce overall calorie intake, and aid in weight management.

4. Bone Health: Some proteins contribute to bone health by helping the body absorb calcium and other minerals necessary for bone strength and density.

5. Repair and Recovery: After illness, injury, or surgery, the body requires additional protein to repair tissues and support recovery.

Common Misconceptions

1. Protein Overconsumption: While protein is crucial, many people overestimate their protein needs, leading to imbalanced diets. Excessive protein intake can strain the kidneys and potentially lead to health issues, especially in those with pre-existing kidney conditions.

2. Protein Sources: There's a misconception that animal products are the only or best protein sources. While animal products like meat, poultry, fish, eggs, and dairy are rich in protein, plant-based sources like beans, lentils, tofu, tempeh, nuts, and seeds also provide ample protein.

3. Muscle Building: While protein is essential for muscle growth, consuming excessive amounts won't necessarily result in bigger muscles. Muscle growth also depends on factors like exercise, overall diet, and individual physiology.

Foods to Eat

1. Animal Sources: Lean meats like chicken, turkey, and fish are excellent sources of high-quality protein. Eggs and dairy products like Greek yogurt and cottage cheese are also protein-rich options.

2. Plant-Based Sources: Legumes such as beans, lentils, chickpeas, and peas are rich in protein and fiber. Tofu, tempeh, edamame, and other soy products are complete protein sources suitable for vegetarians and vegans. Nuts, seeds, quinoa, and whole grains like oats and brown rice contribute to protein intake.

3. Combination Foods: Many foods combine multiple protein sources. For example, peanut butter on whole-grain bread, rice, and beans, or yogurt with nuts and fruit can provide a well-rounded protein boost.

4. Supplementation: Protein supplements like whey protein powder or plant-based protein powders can be convenient options for individuals who struggle to meet their protein needs through whole foods alone. However, whole food sources should remain the primary focus of the diet.

Balancing protein intake with other macronutrients and maintaining a diverse diet is critical to reaping protein benefits while avoiding potential pitfalls.

5

Fats

The fear of fats has persisted for years, but not all fats are harmful. Healthy fats (such as those found in avocados, nuts, and olive oil) are essential for brain health, hormone balance, and overall well-being. Fat-free or low-fat products are often marketed as healthier options; however, these products may contain added sugars or artificial additives to compensate for the lack of flavor.

Importance of Fat

Fats play a crucial role in nutrient absorption and cellular structure. They provide more than two times the number of calories per gram compared to carbohydrates and serve as a basis for hormone production.

1. Fats are essential for absorbing fat-soluble vitamins (A, D, E, and K). Without an adequate intake of dietary fats, the body may struggle to absorb these crucial vitamins, which play roles in immune function, bone health, vision, and more.

2. Cellular Structure: Fats are integral components of cell membranes, contributing to cell structure, flexibility, and integrity. They help regulate what enters and exits cells, ensuring proper cellular

function.

3. Energy Source: Fat is a concentrated energy source, providing more than twice the number of calories per gram compared to carbohydrates or protein. It serves as a long-term energy reserve, particularly during periods of low food intake or endurance activities.

4. Hormone Production: Fats are precursors to various hormones and signaling molecules in the body. Hormones derived from fats play roles in metabolism, reproduction, stress response, and inflammation regulation.

5. Brain Health: The brain is composed primarily of fat, and dietary fats are crucial for brain development, cognitive function, and mood regulation. Omega-3 fatty acids, in particular, are linked to improved brain health and may help reduce the risk of neurodegenerative diseases.

Common Misconceptions

1. All Fats are Bad: One of the most pervasive misconceptions is that all fats are unhealthy. In reality, fats are a diverse group of nutrients; not all fats are created equal. While trans fats and excessive saturated fats are detrimental to health, unsaturated fats, predominantly monounsaturated and polyunsaturated fats, are beneficial and essential for optimal health.

2. Fats Make You Fat: Another misconception is that eating fats leads to weight gain. While fats are energy-dense, consuming them appropriately as part of a balanced diet does not inherently cause weight gain. Excess calorie intake contributes to weight gain regardless of the macronutrient source.

3. Low-Fat is Always Better: Many low-fat or fat-free products are marketed as healthier alternatives. However, these products often

contain added sugars, preservatives, and other additives to compensate for the loss of flavor and texture. Moreover, some essential nutrients are fat-soluble, requiring dietary fat for absorption.

Foods to Eat

1. Healthy Oils: Olive oil, avocado oil, coconut oil, and flaxseed oil are excellent sources of healthy fats, mainly monounsaturated and polyunsaturated fats. These oils can be used for cooking, salad dressings, or as a topping for dishes.
2. Fatty Fish: Salmon, mackerel, trout, sardines, and herring are rich in omega-3 fatty acids, which have been linked to numerous health benefits, including heart health and brain function.
3. Nuts and Seeds: Almonds, walnuts, pecans, chia seeds, flaxseeds, and hemp seeds are packed with healthy fats, protein, fiber, vitamins, and minerals. They make for convenient and nutritious snacks or additions to meals.
4. Avocado: Avocado is a nutrient-dense fruit loaded with heart-healthy monounsaturated fats. It can be sliced, mashed as guacamole, or added to salads, sandwiches, and smoothies.
5. Whole Eggs: Despite misconceptions about their cholesterol content, they are nutritious and provide healthy fats, high-quality protein, vitamins, and minerals. They can be prepared in various ways, such as boiled, scrambled, or as an ingredient in dishes.

Incorporating a variety of healthy fats into your diet can support overall health and well-being. To maintain a balanced diet, consuming fats from natural, whole-food sources and moderate intake is essential.

6

Micronutrients

Your body needs macronutrients and micronutrients, but they are needed in smaller quantities. These elements include vitamins, minerals, iron, and fluoride.

Vitamins are essential for life, and taking small amounts daily is sufficient. Vitamins are consumed from the outside; our bodies do not produce them. The four common elements in all living cells are carbon, hydrogen, oxygen, and nitrogen. Together, these elements make up about 99% of cell masses. Minerals are found in the skeleton and tooth structure; iron and cobalt are important for blood production, and zinc is important for the immune system.

Importance of Micronutrients

1. Nutrient Absorption and Utilization: Micronutrients play crucial roles in facilitating the absorption and utilization of macronutrients (carbohydrates, proteins, and fats). For example, vitamin D is necessary for calcium absorption, while magnesium is involved in hundreds of enzymatic reactions in the body.

2. Cellular Function and Structure: Micronutrients are integral to various cellular functions and structures. They act as cofactors (required for the enzyme to work) for enzymes, antioxidants, and structural components of cells, tissues, and organs. For instance, iron is essential for the formation of hemoglobin, which transports oxygen in the blood.

3. Immune Function: Many micronutrients, such as vitamins A, C, D, and zinc, play vital roles in supporting immune function. They help regulate immune responses, enhance the body's ability to fight infections and promote tissue repair and healing.

4. Energy Production: Micronutrients are involved in energy metabolism, helping convert food into energy the body can use. B vitamins, for example, play critical roles in carbohydrate, fat, and protein metabolism, ensuring efficient energy production.

5. Bone Health: Certain micronutrients, including calcium, vitamin D, vitamin K, and magnesium, are essential for bone health. They contribute to bone formation, density, and strength, reducing the risk of osteoporosis and fractures.

Common Misconceptions

1. Supplements Are Sufficient: Many believe dietary supplements can adequately meet micronutrient needs. While supplements can benefit individuals with specific deficiencies or dietary restrictions, they should not replace a balanced diet rich in micronutrient-dense foods. Whole foods provide a wide array of nutrients in their natural forms, along with other beneficial compounds like fiber and phytonutrients.

2. More Is Better: Some assume excessive micronutrients will enhance health or performance. However, excessive intake of specific vitamins and minerals can be harmful and may lead to toxicity

or adverse health effects. It's essential to meet recommended intake levels without exceeding tolerable upper intake levels (ULs) established for safety.

3. All Foods Are Created Equal: Not all foods contain the same levels of micronutrients. Processed and refined foods often lack essential vitamins, minerals, and other nutrients found in whole, unprocessed foods. Choosing nutrient-dense foods like fruits, vegetables, whole grains, lean proteins, and healthy fats is essential for meeting micronutrient needs.

Foods to Eat

1. Fruits and Vegetables: Aim to include a variety of colorful fruits and vegetables in your diet to ensure a broad spectrum of vitamins, minerals, and antioxidants. Examples include leafy greens, berries, citrus fruits, carrots, bell peppers, and cruciferous vegetables like broccoli and cauliflower.

2. Whole Grains: Opt for whole grains like oats, brown rice, quinoa, barley, and whole wheat, which provide fiber, vitamins (such as B vitamins), minerals (such as magnesium and iron), and phytonutrients.

3. Lean Proteins: Choose lean protein sources like poultry, fish, tofu, legumes, and low-fat dairy products. These foods provide protein and essential micronutrients such as iron, zinc, and B vitamins.

4. Healthy Fats: Incorporate sources of healthy fats like nuts, seeds, avocado, and olive oil into your diet. These foods provide vitamins (such as vitamin E), minerals (such as magnesium), and essential fatty acids like omega-3s.

5. Dairy and Dairy Alternatives: Include dairy products like milk, yogurt, and cheese or fortified dairy alternatives like almond milk and soy milk to obtain calcium, vitamin D, and other micronutrients

important for bone health.

Focusing on a varied and balanced diet that includes a wide range of nutrient-dense foods can ensure adequate intake of essential vitamins, minerals, and other micronutrients necessary for optimal health and function.

7

What About Calorie Count?

Counting calories can be a valuable tool for weight management, but as mentioned earlier, focusing solely on calorie counting may lead to unintended consequences.

Pros of Counting Calories

1. Awareness and Accountability: Counting calories increases awareness of food choices and portion sizes, promoting accountability for dietary intake. It provides a concrete method for tracking energy balance and identifying areas for improvement in nutritional habits.

2. Weight Loss or Maintenance: For many people, consuming fewer calories than they expend can lead to weight loss or help maintain a healthy weight. Counting calories allows individuals to create a calorie deficit necessary for fat loss when combined with other healthy lifestyle habits.

3. Flexibility: Calorie counting allows for flexibility in food choices as long as overall calorie intake aligns with weight management goals. It can accommodate various dietary preferences and restrictions,

empowering individuals to make informed choices while enjoying a wide range of foods.

4. Educational Tool: Counting calories can be a valuable educational tool. It helps individuals learn about the energy content of different foods and the relationship between calorie intake and weight outcomes. This knowledge can contribute to long-term behavior change and improved dietary habits.

Cons of Counting Calories

1. Focus on Quantity Over Quality: Relying solely on calorie counting may prioritize quantity (calories) over quality (nutrient density) of food choices. Some individuals may opt for low-calorie, highly pro-cessed foods over nutrient-rich whole foods, leading to potential nutrient deficiencies and poor overall health.

2. Emotional Impact: Constantly tracking and restricting calories can lead to feelings of anxiety, guilt, or obsession around food. This rigid approach to eating may contribute to disordered eating patterns, including binge eating, yo-yo dieting, or orthorexia, which is an eating disorder focused on eating foods that are perceived as clean, pure, or natural (ignoring entire food groups).

3. Inaccuracy and Variability: Calorie counting relies on estimates of energy content, which can be imprecise and subject to variability. Factors such as cooking methods, food preparation, and individ-ual metabolism can influence calorie absorption and utilization, making it challenging to achieve precise calorie targets.

4. Sustainability and Long-Term Success: Strict calorie counting may not be sustainable in the long term, leading to frustration, burnout, and eventual relapse into old habits. Moreover, weight loss achieved through calorie restriction alone may be challenging to maintain unless underlying lifestyle factors and behaviors are

addressed.

Unintended Consequences

1. Nutrient Imbalance: Focusing solely on calorie counting may result in nutrient imbalances or deficiencies if dietary choices prioritize low-calorie processed foods over nutrient-dense whole foods. Inadequate intake of essential vitamins, minerals, and other nutrients can negatively impact overall health and well-being.

2. Negative Relationship with Food: Obsessive calorie counting can lead to a negative relationship with food, viewing it solely as a source of calories rather than nourishment and enjoyment. This mindset can diminish the pleasure of eating and undermine social interactions centered around food.

3. Disordered Eating Patterns: Strict calorie counting may contribute to disordered eating patterns, including restrictive eating, binge eating, or compulsive exercise. These behaviors can have severe physical and psychological consequences, impairing quality of life and overall health.

4. Metabolic Adaptation: Prolonged calorie restriction may lead to metabolic adaptation, where the body adjusts to lower calorie intake by slowing down metabolism and conserving energy. This can hinder weight loss efforts and make it challenging to achieve sustainable results.

In summary, while counting calories can be a helpful tool for weight management, it's important to approach it with caution and balance. Combining calorie awareness with a focus on nutrient-dense foods, mindful eating practices, and overall lifestyle factors is key to achieving sustainable and holistic health outcomes.

8

Counting Macros - The Basics

While gaining popularity over recent years, counting macronutrients is not necessarily a new diet fad. This approach involves tracking the intake of the three primary macronutrients, carbohydrates, proteins, and fats, to achieve specific ratios or absolute amounts tailored to individual needs.

Factors contributing to the increased interest in this method of weight management

1. Personalization: Counting macros allows for a personalized approach to nutrition, considering individual goals, preferences, and dietary needs. Unlike one-size-fits-all diets, macro counting can be adjusted to accommodate various lifestyles, activity levels, and metabolic differences.
2. Focus on Nutrient Balance: Instead of solely focusing on calories, counting macros emphasizes the balance of macronutrients, ensuring adequate intake of proteins, carbohydrates, and fats. This approach promotes a more balanced and sustainable approach to eating, optimizing nutrient intake for overall health and perfor-

mance.

3. Flexibility: Counting macros offers flexibility in food choices as long as they fit within the prescribed macronutrient targets. This flexibility allows individuals to enjoy a wide variety of foods while still working towards their health and fitness goals, making it more sustainable than restrictive diets.

4. Performance Enhancement: For athletes and fitness enthusiasts, tracking macros can be beneficial for optimizing performance, supporting muscle growth and recovery, and fueling workouts effectively. By fine-tuning macronutrient intake, individuals can tailor their nutrition to meet the demands of their training regimen.

Pros of Counting Macronutrients

1. Precision: Counting macros provides a precise method for monitoring dietary intake, allowing individuals to control their macronutrient ratios and adjust as needed to achieve specific goals, whether it's weight loss, muscle gain, or improved athletic performance.

2. Education and Awareness: Macro counting promotes greater awareness of food choices and their nutritional content. It encourages individuals to learn about the macronutrient composition of different foods and how they impact energy levels, hunger, and satiety.

3. Customization: Macro counting allows for customization based on individual needs and preferences. It can accommodate various dietary restrictions, food preferences, and lifestyle factors, providing a flexible approach to nutrition.

4. Supports Diverse Goals: Whether the goal is weight loss, muscle gain, improved athletic performance, or overall health, counting macros can be adapted to support diverse goals and objectives, making it a versatile approach to nutrition.

Cons of Counting Macronutrients

1. Time and Effort: Counting macros requires time and effort to track food intake, weigh or measure portions, and calculate macronutrient values. This level of detail may be impractical or unsustainable for some individuals, leading to frustration or disengagement.

2. Potential Obsession: Similar to calorie counting, macro tracking can become obsessive for some individuals, leading to an unhealthy fixation on numbers and food. This obsession may contribute to anxiety, stress, or disordered eating behaviors.

3. Focus on Quantity Over Quality: While counting macros emphasizes macronutrient balance, it may overlook the importance of food quality and nutrient density. Focusing solely on hitting macro targets without considering food sources can lead to nutrient imbalances or deficiencies.

4. Not Always Sustainable: For some people, counting macros may not be sustainable in the long term, especially if it feels overly restrictive or rigid. Over time, adherence to strict macro targets may decline, leading to fluctuations in dietary habits and potentially regaining lost weight.

9

How to Calculate Macros

To correlate the percentage distribution of carbohydrates, fats, and protein to calorie counts, you first need to understand the energy density of each macronutrient and whether individual activity levels are considered sedentary, moderately active (everyday exercise), or highly active (advanced training). It's essential to adjust macronutrient intake based on individual goals, preferences, and how you respond to different ratios. Monitoring progress and adjusting as needed is critical to optimizing performance, recovery, and overall well-being.

STEP 1: Determine the Percentage Distribution based on your individual needs.

There is a common rule of thumb for macro ratios: 40-30-30. 40% of macros come from carbohydrates, 30% from protein, and 30% from fats. The USDA publishes dietary guidelines and recommendations that can be found at DietaryGuidelines.gov. We are unique with varying activity levels and lifestyles, so you may require a different macro split. Here are some considerations:

Sedentary Individuals

Sedentary individuals typically have low levels of physical activity. They may spend most of their time sitting or engaging in minimal physical activity.

Macronutrient distribution:

- Protein: 10-20% of total daily calories
- Carbohydrates: 45-55% of total daily calories
- Fats: 25-35% of total daily calories

Focusing on whole, nutrient-dense foods and controlling portion sizes may benefit these individuals in maintaining a healthy weight and supporting overall health.

Moderately Active (Everyday Exercise):

The "everyday athlete" engages in regular physical activity or exercise several times a week, such as recreational sports, jogging, or fitness classes.

Macronutrient distribution:

- Protein: 20-25% of total daily calories
- Carbohydrates: 50-55% of total daily calories
- Fats: 20-30% of total daily calories

These individuals require slightly higher protein intake to support muscle repair and recovery, along with sufficient carbohydrates for energy during workouts and fats for overall health.

Highly Active (Advanced Exercise):

Advanced athletes regularly participate in intense training or competitive sports and may have high energy expenditure.

Macronutrient distribution:

- Protein: 25-35% of total daily calories
- Carbohydrates: 55-65% of total daily calories
- Fats: 20-30% of total daily calories

These individuals need more protein and carbohydrates to support muscle maintenance, repair, and energy production during intense training sessions. Adequate fat intake is also important for hormone regulation and overall health.

STEP TWO: Determine Your Total Energy Expended Daily

It's important to know where to begin with your caloric intake. Here are some acronyms that are used throughout this discussion which you should become familiar with:

Total Energy Expenditure (TEE) = REE + NREE. This total represents the calories your body needs over 24 hours to maintain weight. TEE includes both the Resting Energy Expenditure and Non-Resting Energy Expenditure.

Resting Energy Expenditure (REE) represents the energy your body needs at rest and accounts for about *70% of your TEE* (what you burn when your body is resting). This is also commonly referred to as Resting Metabolic Rate.

Non-Resting Energy Expenditure (NREE) includes calories burned through non-physical activity and the thermodynamic effect of food (TEF). It is approximately *30% of your TEE*. Interestingly, exercise accounts for about 5% of your TEE, which really points to the critical fact that most of the energy expenditure does not stem from exercise alone. If your goal is to lose weight, exercise shouldn't be your primary focus.

Thermic Effect of Food (TEF) constitutes approximately 10% of your TEE (included in NREE). When you consume food, your body needs energy to digest, absorb, transport, and metabolize the nutrients from that food. Macronutrients play a crucial role here as different macronutrients have varying thermic effects. Protein has the highest thermic effect, followed by carbohydrates and fats.

Physical Activity Level (PAL) is a factor used to measure a person's physical activity level by comparing their energy usage over 24 hours to the energy needed to keep the body at rest.

Calculating your total energy expenditure (TEE) involves estimating both your resting energy expenditure (REE) and your non-resting energy expenditure (NREE).

Here is an easy online calculator to save you all the trouble of doing math: https://tdeecalculator.net/

For those who want to calculate each component yourself, here's the formulas and calculation examples:

Resting Energy Expenditure (REE)

There are several equations commonly used to estimate REE, with the Mifflin-St Jeor equation being one of the most widely used and validated methods. The formula for estimating REE is as follows:

For men: REE = (10 × weight in kg) + (6.25 × height in cm) − (5 × age in years) + 5

For women: REE = (10 × weight in kg) + (6.25 × height in cm) - (5 × age in years) − 161

Examples

Note: To convert pounds to kilograms, divide the number of pounds by 2.2; convert inches to centimeters by multiplying the inch value by 2.54.

For a 200-pound male, 6 ft. tall, 50 years old
REE = (10 x 91 kg) + (6.25 x 183 cm) − (5 x 50) + 5 = 1808

For a 150-pound female, 5'-6" ft. tall, 50 years old
REE = (10 x 68 kg) + (6.25 x 167.6 cm) − (5 x 50) - 161 = 1316.5

Once you calculate your REE using one of these equations, you'll have an estimate of the number of calories your body needs at rest to maintain basic physiological functions such as breathing, circulation, and cell repair.

Non-Resting Energy Expenditure (NREE)

Non-resting energy expenditure includes the calories burned through physical activity and the thermic effect of food (TEF).

Total Energy Expenditure (TEE)

The TEE includes both the REE and the NREE. To calculate, simply multiply the REE by an appropriate Physical Activity Level (PAL) factor. This factor is based on your activity level throughout the day. PAL values typically range from sedentary (PAL ≈ 1.2) to highly active (PAL ≈ 2.4).

- Little to no exercise – a desk job and minimal physical activity outside of work: 1.2
- Light activity – walking, yoga, leisurely biking, 30 minutes, 1-3 days a week: 1.375
- Moderate activity – jogging, swimming, weight training, 30 minutes to 1 hour 3-5 days per week: 1.55
- Active – challenging exercise such as intense training or competitive sports, 1-2 hours on 6-7 days per week: 1.725
- Very active – tough exercise, sports, physical job, or training twice per day, such as marathon training or heavy lifting: 1.9 or higher

To estimate TEE, multiply your REE by your PAL: TEE = REE x PAL

Using the above example:

For Men: If your PAL reflects Moderate activity.
   TEE = 1808 x 1.55 = 2802

For Women: If your PAL reflects Moderate activity.
   TEE = 1316.5 x 1.55 = 2040 example

This represents the approximate number of calories you expend through physical activity, the thermic effect of food each day, and your resting energy expenditure.

Additionally, you can track calories burned through exercise using activity trackers, heart rate monitors, or online calculators to get a more accurate estimate of your NREE.

How to Calculate the Macronutrient Calories based on your Total Energy Expenditure (TEE)

You can easily calculate caloric value when reading nutrition labels or weighing foods such as meats.

Carbohydrates

- To calculate the calorie contribution of carbohydrates, multiply the percentage distribution of carbohydrates by the total calorie intake.
- Example: If you're consuming 2000 calories per day and want 40% of those calories to come from carbohydrates:
- Calories from Carbohydrates = (0.40×2000) = 800 calories
- Carbohydrates provide approximately 4 calories per gram.

Protein

- To calculate protein's calorie contribution, multiply the protein percentage distribution by the total calorie intake.
- Example: Using the same 2000 calorie per day example, if you want 30% of those calories to come from protein:
- Calories from Protein = (0.30×2000) = 600 calories
- Protein also provides approximately 4 calories per gram.

Fats

- To calculate the calorie contribution of fats, multiply the percentage distribution of fats by the total calorie intake.
- Example: Using the same 2000 calorie per day example, if you want 30% of those calories to come from fats:
- Calories from Fats = (0.30×2000) = 600 calories

- Fats are more energy-dense and provide approximately 9 calories per gram.

After calculating the calorie contributions of each macronutrient, you can verify that they add up to the total calorie intake for the day. In this example: 800 calories from Carbohydrates + 600 calories from Protein + 600 calories from Fats = 2000 total calories

This approach allows you to establish the desired percentage distribution of macronutrients within your total calorie intake and ensure that your diet aligns with your nutritional goals.

When adjusting macronutrient intake based on activity level and energy expenditure, a general rule of thumb is maintaining the same percentage distribution of macronutrients but adjusting the total calorie intake to accommodate the increased energy needs. However, there are some considerations to keep in mind:

1. Maintain Relative Macronutrient Ratios: If you have established a specific percentage distribution of carbohydrates, proteins, and fats that aligns with your goals and preferences, you can maintain these ratios even as your calorie intake fluctuates. For example, if you're increasing your activity level and calorie intake to support higher energy expenditure, aim to maintain the same percentage of calories from carbohydrates, proteins, and fats.

2. Adjust Total Caloric Intake: As your energy expenditure increases due to higher activity levels, you'll need to consume more calories to meet your energy needs and prevent weight loss. Adjust your total calorie intake upward based on your estimated energy expenditure while keeping the percentage distribution of macronutrients consistent.

3. Consider Timing and Composition: While the overall percentage distribution of macronutrients may remain constant, you may choose to adjust the timing and composition of meals to support your activity level. For example, increase carbohydrate intake before and after workouts to fuel performance and enhance recovery.

4. Individual Variation: Remember that individual responses to changes in activity level and macronutrient intake can vary. Some individuals may find that they perform better with slightly higher carbohydrate intake. In contrast, others may prefer a higher proportion of fats or protein. Experimentation and monitoring of performance, energy levels, and body composition can help determine the optimal macronutrient distribution for your needs.

In summary, when adjusting macronutrient intake based on activity level and energy expenditure, aim to maintain the same relative distribution of carbohydrates, proteins, and fats while adjusting total calorie intake to support increased energy needs. Monitor your progress and adjust to optimize performance, recovery, and overall health.

A final note: Even on rest days, you want to maintain consistency in your macro percentages. Do not decrease your macros. While you do not have as much physical activity, this is when your muscles are repairing and rebuilding, and the best way to aid this process is with food.

10

Body Types and Macronutrient Counting

ody type, or somatotype, can somewhat influence macronutrient needs and preferences. The term "somatotype" refers
to a classification system that describes and categorizes
an individual's body shape or physique based on certain physical
characteristics. It was developed by American psychologist William
H. Sheldon in the 1940s. Sheldon proposed three primary somatotypes
or body types, each associated with specific physical traits and potential
personality characteristics.

Sheldon's somatotype theory suggested that an individual's body type
influences their physical appearance and correlates with certain personality traits and predispositions. For example, he proposed that
mesomorphs are more likely to be assertive, competitive, and dominant,
while ectomorphs may be more introverted, sensitive, and intellectual,
and endomorphs may exhibit traits such as sociability and relaxation.

While Sheldon's somatotype theory has been criticized for its lack of
scientific rigor and oversimplification of human variation, the concept
of somatotypes continues to be used informally to describe general body

shapes and characteristics. However, it's essential to recognize that human bodies are diverse, and individuals may not neatly fit into one of Sheldon's categories. Additionally, personality traits are influenced by many factors beyond physical appearance.

Here are the **three somatotypes** briefly describing how they influence macronutrient needs.

Ectomorphs: Individuals with a naturally lean and slender build may have higher carbohydrate requirements to fuel their fast metabolism and support energy needs, particularly if they're highly active or have a speedy metabolism.

- Macronutrient Distribution: A balanced macronutrient distribution might include around 40-50% of calories from carbohydrates, 25-30% from protein, and 25-30% from fats.
- Protein: Aim for a moderate to high protein intake to support muscle growth and repair. Include lean protein sources such as chicken, turkey, fish, tofu, legumes, and low-fat dairy.
- Carbohydrates: Prioritize complex carbohydrates from whole grains, fruits, vegetables, and legumes to provide sustained energy and support athletic performance.
- Fats: Include healthy fats from sources like nuts, seeds, avocados, and olive oil to provide essential fatty acids and support overall health.

Mesomorphs: Those with a mesomorphic body type, characterized by a muscular and athletic build, may benefit from a balanced macronutrient ratio, including adequate protein to support muscle growth and repair, along with sufficient carbohydrates for energy.

- Macronutrient Distribution: A balanced macronutrient distribution might include around 30-40% of calories from carbohydrates, 30-40% from protein, and 20-30% from fats.
- Protein: Aim for a moderate to high protein intake to support muscle growth, repair, and recovery. Include a variety of protein sources, both animal and plant-based, to ensure adequate amino acid intake.
- Carbohydrates: Consume complex carbohydrates from whole grains, fruits, vegetables, and legumes to provide energy for workouts and support glycogen replenishment.
- Fats: Include healthy fats in moderation to support hormone production, satiety, and overall health. Choose sources like nuts, seeds, avocados, and fatty fish.

Endomorphs: Endomorphs, who tend to have a higher body fat percentage and a slower metabolism, may benefit from a macronutrient distribution that prioritizes protein and healthy fats to promote satiety and stabilize blood sugar levels while moderating carbohydrate intake to manage weight.

- Macronutrient Distribution: Aim for around 25-35% of calories from carbohydrates, 30-40% from protein, and 30-35% from fats.
- Protein: Emphasize a higher protein intake to support satiety, muscle preservation, and metabolic rate. Include lean protein sources and consider spacing protein intake evenly throughout the day.
- Carbohydrates: Focus on moderate carbohydrate intake from nutrient-dense sources like vegetables, fruits, and whole grains. Pay attention to portion sizes and choose carbohydrates with a lower glycemic index to help manage blood sugar levels.
- Fats: Include healthy fats to support satiety, hormone production, and nutrient absorption. Choose sources like nuts, seeds, avocados,

olive oil, and moderate intake to support weight management goals.

When devising a plan for counting macros based on somatotype, it's essential to consider individual differences in metabolism, body composition, activity level, and goals. While somatotype can provide a general framework for understanding body types, it's not the sole determinant of macronutrient needs.

11

Maximize Benefits - Sustainability

To sustain macronutrient counting long-term and see lasting improvements in health and fitness, here are some practical tips and advice:

1. Focus on Balance and Variety: Aim for a balanced diet that includes a variety of nutrient-dense foods from all food groups. Include a variety of fruits, vegetables, whole grains, lean proteins, and healthy fats to ensure you're meeting your nutritional needs.

2. Build Sustainable Habits: Instead of viewing macronutrient counting as a short-term diet, approach it as a long-term lifestyle change. Build sustainable habits around mindful eating, portion control, and balanced nutrition that you can maintain for the long haul. Consistency and adherence to healthy habits over time are key to achieving lasting results.

3. Gradual Progression: Start with small, manageable changes rather than trying to overhaul your entire diet overnight. Gradually incorporate macro counting into your routine and experiment with different approaches to find the best for you. Start with protein, and once you feel confident eating the right amount of protein, dial

in your carbs and fats. Focus on making incremental improvements over time rather than striving for perfection from the outset.

4. Listen to Your Body: Pay attention to hunger and satiety cues, energy levels, and how different foods make you feel. Use macro counting to become more mindful of your dietary choices and how they impact your overall well-being. Adjust your approach based on feedback from your body. Protein will help you feel fuller and have more energy. Fats should be avoided around workouts as they are digested more quickly than carbs, and carbs are the primary fuel your body consumes during workouts.

5. Flexibility and Adaptability: Be flexible and adaptable in your approach to macro counting. Life circumstances, preferences, and goals may change over time, so be willing to adjust your macro targets and dietary habits accordingly. Allow yourself to enjoy occasional treats or deviations from your usual routine without guilt, focusing on overall balance and moderation.

6. Seek Support and Accountability: Surround yourself with a supportive network of friends, family, or online communities who share similar health and fitness goals. Accountability partners can help keep you motivated, encourage you during challenging times, and offer valuable insights and tips for sustaining macro counting long-term.

7. Celebrate Non-Scale Victories: While tracking progress on the scale can be motivating, remember to celebrate non-scale victories as well. Focus on improvements in energy levels, strength, endurance, mood, and overall well-being, which are often more meaningful indicators of success than changes in body weight alone.

By adopting a balanced, flexible, and sustainable approach to macro counting, you can incorporate this practice into your lifestyle long-term and reap the benefits of improved health, fitness, and overall well-being.

Remember that consistency, patience, and self-compassion are key to long-term success on your health journey.

How to Navigate "Those" Days

Experiencing a day where you deviate from your macronutrient counting plan and eat in a way that feels "crazy" or unplanned is a shared experience, and it's important to approach it with kindness and self-compassion. Here's some advice to help you navigate those moments:

1. Don't Beat Yourself Up: It's natural to feel disappointed or frustrated when you veer off track, but it's essential to practice self-compassion and avoid harsh self-criticism. Remind yourself that one day of overindulgence does not undo all of your progress and doesn't define your worth or success.

2. Avoid All-or-Nothing Thinking: Instead of viewing one off-plan day as a failure, reframe it as a temporary setback or learning opportunity. Recognize that dietary adherence is not black and white, and it's expected to have occasional deviations from your plan. What matters most is your overall consistency and commitment to your health goals over time.

3. Reflect on Triggers and Patterns: Use moments of deviation as an opportunity for self-reflection. Identify any triggers or patterns that may have contributed to the unplanned eating, such as stress, boredom, emotional triggers, or social situations. Understanding your triggers can help you develop strategies to address them more effectively in the future.

4. Practice Mindful Eating: Cultivate awareness and mindfulness around your eating habits, particularly during moments of impulsivity or emotional eating. Pause and check in before reaching for food, asking yourself if you're starving or if other underlying

emotions or needs drive your desire to eat.

5. Recommit to Your Goals: Rather than dwelling on the past, focus on the present moment and recommit to your health and fitness goals. Remind yourself why you started macro counting in the first place and the positive changes you've experienced along the way. Use your commitment as motivation to get back on track and make healthier choices moving forward.

6. Plan for the Future: Take proactive steps to prevent future instances of unplanned eating by planning ahead and creating strategies for managing challenging situations. This could involve meal prepping, stocking your pantry with healthy options, practicing stress-reduction techniques, or seeking support from friends, family, or a coach.

7. Practice Forgiveness and Let Go: Finally, practice forgiveness, both for yourself and for any perceived mistakes or shortcomings. Let go of guilt and self-judgment, and instead, focus on the present moment and the positive steps you can take to support your health and well-being moving forward.

Remember that consistency and progress are more important than perfection. Embrace the journey, celebrate your successes, and be gentle with yourself during moments of challenge or setback. Every day is an opportunity to make choices that align with your values and support your long-term health and happiness.

12

Mindset Matters

Mindset plays a crucial role in successfully making a change in your life, including adopting practices like counting macronutrients for nutrition, weight loss, or bodybuilding, for several reasons:

1. Motivation and Commitment: A positive mindset can fuel motivation and commitment to your goals. When you believe in your ability to succeed and visualize the benefits of your efforts, you're more likely to stay dedicated to your nutrition plan, even when faced with challenges or setbacks.

2. Resilience and Persistence: A growth-oriented mindset encourages resilience and persistence in facing obstacles. Instead of viewing setbacks as failures, you see them as opportunities for growth and learning. This resilience helps you bounce back from setbacks and stay on track toward your goals.

3. Self-Efficacy: Mindset influences your self-efficacy, or belief in your ability to succeed. When you have a confident mindset, you're more likely to tackle challenges with determination and view setbacks as temporary setbacks rather than insurmountable

obstacles. This belief in your own capabilities empowers you to take action and overcome barriers to success.

4. Adaptability and Flexibility: A growth mindset promotes adaptability and flexibility in your approach to change. Instead of rigidly adhering to a specific plan or outcome, you're open to trying new strategies, learning from feedback, and adjusting your approach. This flexibility allows you to find what works best for you and make sustainable changes over time.

5. Positive Habits and Behaviors: Mindset influences your habits and behaviors related to nutrition and health. When you cultivate a positive mindset, you're more likely to engage in behaviors that support your goals, such as planning meals, prioritizing nutrient-dense foods, practicing mindful eating, and staying consistent with your macronutrient tracking.

6. Emotional Well-being: A positive mindset promotes emotional well-being and resilience, essential for navigating the ups and downs of behavior change. When you approach your nutrition journey with a positive attitude and self-compassion, you're better equipped to manage stress, overcome setbacks, and maintain a healthy relationship with food and your body.

7. Long-Term Success: Ultimately, mindset can determine your long-term success in making sustainable changes to your nutrition, weight, and fitness. By cultivating a growth-oriented mindset and focusing on the process of change rather than just the outcome, you set yourself up for lasting success and well-being.

In summary, mindset matters when it comes to successfully making a change in your life, like counting macronutrients for nutrition, weight loss, or bodybuilding. It influences your motivation, resilience, self-efficacy, adaptability, habits, emotional well-being, and long-term success. By cultivating a positive and growth-oriented mindset, you can overcome obstacles, stay committed to your goals, and create lasting changes that support your health and happiness.

13

Key Takeaways

Counting macros is about finding what works best for you. When you have the right tools and knowledge, you can manage your diet successfully and sustain it well into the future. It is important to be flexible. Tracking your results is important so you can adjust along the way. As you have periods of lower activity or higher activity, you now know how to modify your calories and macros accordingly.

Whole, minimally processed foods retain more nutrients and health-promoting compounds than highly processed or refined foods, which may be stripped of nutrients and contain added sugars, unhealthy fats, and preservatives. Choose whole, unprocessed foods whenever possible.

When planning a balanced diet, it's essential to consider foods' overall nutritional profile beyond their calorie content. By focusing on a variety of nutrient-dense foods rich in macronutrients, micronutrients, and fiber, you can optimize your nutrition, support overall health and well-being, and enhance your long-term vitality.

Finally, consider consulting with a registered dietitian or nutritionist for personalized guidance and support in devising a macro counting plan tailored to your somatotype, goals, and lifestyle. They can provide individualized recommendations and help you navigate any challenges or questions that arise along the way.

14

References

Davis, S. (2024, February 19). Top nutrition and fitness trends in 2024, according to experts. *Forbes Health.* https://www.forbes.com/health/wellness/top-nutrition-and-fitness-trends-2024/

Essential Foods for Optimal Childhood Nutrition. https://www.technews23.com/2023/08/essential-foods-for-optimal-childhood.htmlHeath, B. H., & Carter, J. E. L. (1967). A modified somatotype method. *American Journal of Physical Anthropology,* 27(1), 57–74. https://doi.org/10.1002/ajpa.1330270108

How to count your macros. (2023, July 10). https://www.crunch.com.au/blog/nutrition-fuel/how-to-count-your-macros-2/. Retrieved May 5, 2024, from https://www.crunch.com.au/blog/nutrition-fuel/how-to-count-your-macros-2/

Know Your Macros—Why Macronutrients are key to healthy eating. (n.d.). https://www.cedars-sinai.org/blog/what-are-macronutrients.html#:~:text=%22Macros%22%20is%20short%20for%20macronutrients,Read

:%20The%20Science%20of%20Eating

Ldn, I. V. R. (2023, January 4). *Should You Be Counting Macros? Here's What a Dietitian Has to Say.* EatingWell. https://www.eatingwell.com/article/8022629/counting-macros/

Nourish Goals – Blog: Understanding Macronutrients – Proteins, Carbohydrates, and Fats. https://nourishgoals.com/NGBlog2023081701

Professional, C. C. M. (n.d.). *Carbohydrates.* Cleveland Clinic. https://my.clevelandclinic.org/health/articles/15416-carbohydrates

Sheldon, W. H. (1940). *The Varieties of Human Physique: An introduction to Constitutional Psychology.* Harper & Brothers.

Tasgin, E. (2017). Macronutrients and Micronutrients in Nutrition. International Journal of Innovative Resesarch and Reviews, 1(1), 10-15.